Sleep and Daily Rhythms

Activities Guide for Teachers

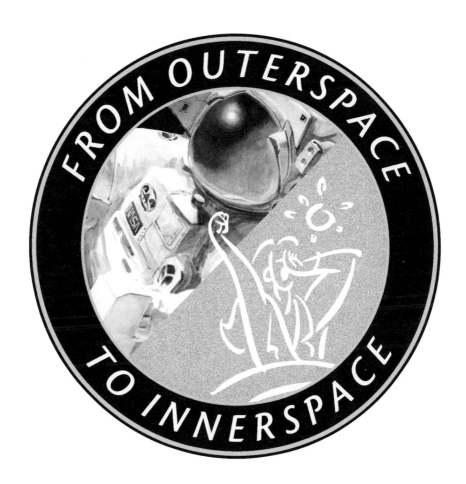

FROM OUTERSPACE

TO INNERSPACE

National Space Biomedical Research Institute
Houston, Texas

The National Space Biomedical Research Institute (NSBRI) is combining the basic research capabilities of some of the nation's leading biomedical research centers with operational and applied research conducted by the National Aeronautics and Space Administration (NASA) to understand and achieve safe and effective long-term human exploration and development of space. The NSBRI's discoveries and research products will help to counter the effects of weightlessness and space radiation and will contribute to the health and well-being of all mankind.

National Space Biomedical Research Institute
One Baylor Plaza, NA-425
Houston, Texas 77030-3498
http://www.nsbri.org

Authors: Nancy P. Moreno, Ph.D. and Barbara Z. Tharp, M.S.
Cover Illustration: T Lewis
Design and Production: Martha S. Young

Acknowledgments
The authors gratefully acknowledge the support of Bobby R. Alford, M.D.; Laurence R. Young, Sc.D.; and Ronald J. White, Ph.D.; as well as the contributions of the following science reviewers: Mary A. Carskadon, Ph.D.; Kimberly Chang, Ph.D.; Charles A. Czeisler, Ph.D., M.D.; David F. Dinges, Ph.D.; Hans P.A. Van Dongen, Ph.D.; and Kenneth P. Wright, Jr., Ph.D. Preparation of this guide would not have been possible without the invaluable assistance of the following field test teachers: Yolanda Adams, Jeri Alloway, Vivian Ashley, Susan Babac, Henrietta Barrera, Paula Clark, Carol Daniels, Barbara Foreman, Carolyn Hopper, Susan King-Martin, Mary Helen Kirby, Sue Klein, Jacqueline McMahon, Sandra Prill, Carol Reams, Mary Ellen Reid, Saundra Saunders, Angi Signorelli, and Marcia Wutke.

The National Aeronautics and Space Administration (NASA) supported this work through the NASA Cooperative Agreement NCC9-58 with the National Space Biomedical Research Institute.

© 2000 by Baylor College of Medicine
All rights reserved. Published 2000
Printed in the United States of America
ISBN: 1-888997-41-9

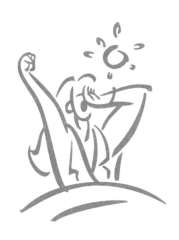

Table of Contents

What Can We Learn in Space

There are many reasons to study life sciences in microgravity, from obvious ones such as ensuring astronaut health to less obvious ones such as improving health care on Earth. The human body is designed to operate in Earth's gravity field. When humans are removed from this environment, as when they travel in space, many complex changes take place: their bones become weaker, fluids shift toward the upper body, body rhythms are disrupted and motion sickness may occur. Life science research allows us to begin planning for long-term stays in space and provides important new medical information that may affect the health care of people here on Earth, such as the ways we care for persons undergoing prolonged bedrest, or those with osteoporosis.

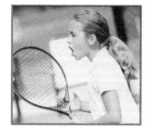

BALANCE. During their first days in space, astronauts can become dizzy and nauseated. Eventually they get over it, but once they return to Earth, they have a hard time walking and standing upright. Finding ways to counteract these changes could benefit millions of Americans with balance disorders.

BONES. Astronauts' bones become weak and porous, because the bones are not working against the Earth's gravity. Many people on Earth, particularly older women, also develop weak bones. Space research on bone will help millions of people with osteoporosis.

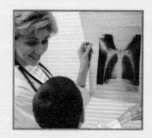

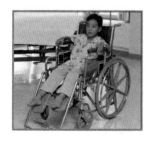

CANCER/RADIATION. Outside the Earth's protective atmosphere, astronauts are exposed to many kinds of damaging radiation that can lead to cell damage and increase astronauts' chances of developing tumors. Learning how to keep astronauts safe from space radiation may improve cancer treatments for people on Earth.

From Outerspace to Innerspace / Sleep and Daily Rhythms
© 2000 Baylor College of Medicine

About Our Bodies Here on Earth?

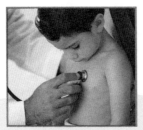

HEART & CIRCULATION. Without gravity, the amount of blood in the body is reduced. The heart becomes smaller and weaker. This becomes a problem when astronauts return to Earth. It makes them feel dizzy and weak. Heart failure and diabetes, experienced by many people on Earth, lead to similar problems.

IMMUNE SYSTEM. It may be easier for astronauts to become sick or develop diseases by living and working in space. Learning about changes in the astronauts' blood and immune systems will help us understand many diseases already here on Earth.

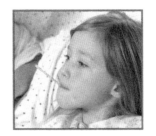

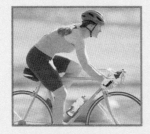

MUSCLES. When muscles do not have to work against gravity, they weaken and begin to waste away. Special exercises and other strategies to help astronauts' muscles stay strong in space also may help older and bedridden people, who experience similar problems on Earth.

SLEEP & WORK. It is hard for astronauts to get enough sleep because the day/night cycle of Earth is lost and there are many distractions. Strategies to help astronauts perform without errors also will benefit people such as airline pilots, or those who must work at night.

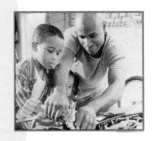

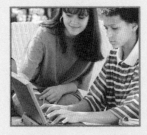

TECHNOLOGY. Special systems and equipment, new diagnostic tools and intelligent computer software that support life science research—as well as the health of astronauts in space—also will improve diagnosis and care for patients on Earth.

Using Cooperative Groups in the Classroom

Cooperative learning is a systematic way for students to work together in groups of two to four. It provides an organized setting for group interaction and enables students to share ideas and to learn from one another. Students in such an environment are more likely to take responsibility for their own learning. The use of cooperative groups provides support for reluctant learners, models community settings where cooperation is necessary, and enables the teacher to conduct hands-on investigations with fewer materials.

Organization is essential for cooperative learning to occur in a hands-on science classroom. Materials must be managed, investigations conducted, results recorded, and clean-up directed and carried out. When a class is "doing" science, each student must have a specific role, or chaos may result.

The Teaming Up! model* provides an efficient system of cooperative learning. Four "jobs" are delineated: Principal Investigator, Materials Manager, Reporter, and Maintenance Director. Each job entails specific responsibilities. Students wear job badges that describe their duties. Tasks are rotated within each group for different activities, so that each student has an opportunity to experience all roles. Teachers even may want to make class charts to coordinate job assignments within groups. For groups with fewer than four students, job assignments can be combined.

Once a cooperative model for learning is established in the classroom, students are able to conduct science activities in an organized and effective manner. All students are aware of their responsibilities and are able to contribute to successful group efforts.

Principal Investigator
Reads the directions
Asks the questions
Checks the work

Materials Manager
Picks up the materials
Uses the equipment
Returns the materials

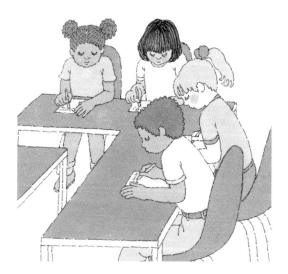

Maintenance Director
Follows the safety rules
Directs the clean up
Asks others to help

Reporter
Writes down observations
and results
Explains the results
Tells the teacher when
the group is finished

* Jones, R.M. 1990. Teaming Up! LaPorte, Texas: ITGROUP.

- The Earth rotates completely on its axis about every 24 hours.
- Cycles of day and night are caused by this rotation and the Earth's position relative to the sun.

OVERVIEW
Students will make a "mini-globe" to discover what makes day and night happen on Earth.

SCIENCE, HEALTH & MATH SKILLS
- Observing
- Measuring
- Modeling
- Mapping
- Drawing conclusions

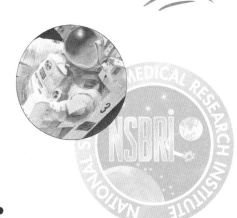

1. What Goes Around . . .

Background

Our lives and those of other organisms on Earth are shaped in countless ways by the cycles of day and night. This repeating pattern of light and darkness is caused by the spinning of our planet and the position of the sun.

Earth, like other planets in our solar system, revolves around the sun in a slightly elliptical orbit. As it does so, the Earth also rotates, or spins, on its axis. It takes about 24 hours for Earth to complete one rotation. As students will discover through the activities in this unit, functions of living organisms are linked to this cycle.

During one 24-hour period, a given location on Earth will experience several hours of sunlight (day time) followed by a period of darkness (night time). One complete rotation equals one day.

As viewed from the North Pole, the Earth spins counterclockwise. This makes the sun appear to come up in the east and to set in the west. In reality, of course, the position of the sun remains relatively constant—while the Earth rotates. The following activity helps students visualize this process through the creation of a simple model. The model will help students understand the Earth's rotation about its axis and the occurrence of day and night. It also will demonstrate the slight tilt in the axis of the Earth.

Time

20 minutes for set-up; 30 minutes to conduct activity

Materials

Each group will need:
- large paper clip
- table tennis (ping-pong) or round foam ball (diameter of 1–2 in.)
- flashlight
- sheet of cardstock (8 1/2 x 11 in.)
- pencils or permanent colored markers
- copy of *Spinning Worlds* page
- copy of *Day & Night* page

Set-up and Management

Before the activity, follow the student instructions on page 4 and make a demonstration "mini-globe," using a ball, paper clip, sheet of card stock and markers.

If using table tennis balls, make a small hole in the bottom of each ball using a push pin before distributing the balls to students. For younger students, you also may want to straighten the paper clip as directed.

Place the materials for each session in a central area for Materials Managers to collect for their groups. Have students work in groups.

Procedure

1. Challenge students to think about what causes night and day to happen

The Earth rotates at a speed of about 1,600 kilometers per hour. Each day on Earth lasts about 24 hours, when measured according to the position of the sun in the sky. Day lengths are different on other planets. One rotation of Mars takes 24.6 Earth hours; one rotation of Jupiter is 9.9 Earth hours; and one rotation of Venus takes 243 Earth days!

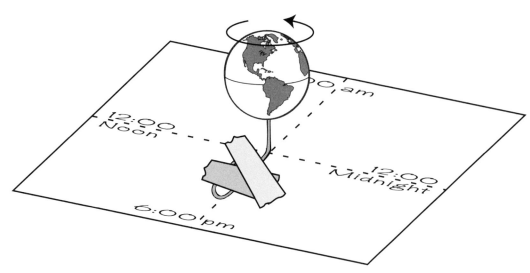

Students will create models of the Earth to understand its rotation.

on Earth. Conduct a discussion and list students' ideas on the board. Challenge their thinking by posing questions such as, *Are days and nights always the same length? Is day always followed by night? Does the sun shine at night? Why does the sun appear in the east in the morning and disappear in the west in the evening? If you add the number of hours in a day to the number of hours in the following night, will the sum always equal 24 hours?* List any additional questions that are posed by students.

2. Tell students that they will be conducting an investigation to help answer many of their questions about day and night on Earth. Explain that each group will construct a small model of the Earth and investigate what happens when light shines on the model.

3. Show the students a mini-globe you have made using a small ball, large paper clip, sheet of card stock and markers (see directions on page 4). The model can be as simple or as elaborate as you choose, depending on

the grade level. Tell students that they will be using similar materials to make their models. Distribute the *Spinning Worlds* directions sheets to students and instruct the Materials Managers to pick up supplies for their groups from a central area.

4. Have students build their models following the instructions given on the *Spinning Worlds* sheet.

5. Once they have completed their models, have students identify which end of the model Earth represents the North Pole. Next, have them determine in which direction the model Earth must spin if it is to rotate in a counterclockwise direction when viewed from above the North Pole. You may need to review *clockwise* and *counterclockwise* for students. Have students stand and face the same direction. Have them turn in place, first clockwise, then counterclockwise.

6. Distribute copies of the *Day & Night* page to each group and have them work through the questions provided.

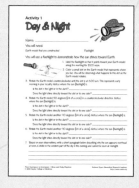

The length of day and night changes throughout the year as a result of the Earth's tilted axis. The axis is the imaginary line that runs from the North Pole through the center of the Earth to the South Pole. If the axis were straight up and down relative to the sun, all days and nights would be 12 hours long throughout the year. However, since the axis is slightly tilted, the hemisphere that leans toward the sun at any given time experiences longer days and shorter nights. That hemisphere also receives more direct rays of light. The combined effect of longer days and more direct light causes the season known as summer.

7. Depending on the ages of your students, you also may want to discuss the effect of the Earth's tilted axis on day length throughout the year, and on the seasons, as described on page two.

8. Ask students to reconsider each of the questions that were asked at the beginning of the activity. Have students use their models to provide the answers. *Are days and nights always the same length?* No, for each location, day and night lengths vary according to the time of year and distance from the equator. *Is day always followed by night?* Yes, in most locations. However, the sun is visible all the time at the poles during the summer season. *Does the sun shine at night?* Yes, the sun always is shining, even though part of the planet is in darkness. Similarly, part of Earth always is facing away and shaded from the sun. *Why does the sun appear in the east in the morning and disappear in the west in the evening?* The direction of rotation of the planet makes the sun appear to rise in the east and to set in the west. *If you add the number of hours in a day to the number of hours in the following night, will the sum always equal 24 hours?* For all locations, except the geographic north and south poles, each day/night cycle equals about 24 hours.

Variations

• Using information available in the newspaper, from weather broadcasts or on the Internet, have students keep a record of the times of sunrise and sunset for several weeks for their locality. If possible, compare the information to times for a location in the Southern Hemisphere.

• Astronauts in orbit circle the Earth every 90 minutes. Have students calculate the number of day/night cycles that a crew of astronauts might experience during a 24-hour period aboard the space shuttle.

• Challenge students to think about why portions of the Arctic are referred to as the "Land of the Midnight Sun." Help them understand that, during summer in the Northern Hemisphere, the North Pole and Arctic regions face toward the sun. This leads to continuous light throughout the day and night periods. Have students think about what happens when the South Pole and Antarctic regions are tilted toward the sun, and what happens to these regions during winter months.

• Discuss with students the effect of the Earth's tilt on the seasons. For example, when it is winter in the Northern Hemisphere, it is summer in the Southern Hemisphere. Give students a list of various cities around the world. Have them predict whether residents of each city would be experiencing winter or summer in July. Next, have students use a globe to locate each city and verify their predictions.

Rotation (turning around a center point or axis) is measured in degrees. A complete rotation is 360°. As seen from the North Pole, the Earth rotates in a counterclockwise direction—or from west to east.

_____

The common abbreviation for morning, a.m., comes from the Latin *ante meridiem*, which means "before noon." The abbreviation, p.m., comes from the Latin *post meridiem*, meaning "after noon."

Activity 1
Spinning Worlds

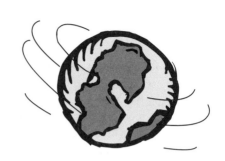

You will need:

Table tennis (ping-pong) or foam ball

Sheet of heavy paper or cardstock

Large paper clip

Colored markers

Make a model of the Earth by following these steps.

1. Fold the heavy paper in half twice. This will make four equal sections. Smooth the sheet and label the folds as shown to the right..

2. Draw a line around the widest part of the ball using a pencil or marker. This represents the equator on your Earth model.

3. Draw the continents on the ball using the diagrams below as guides. Be sure to notice which pole is north and which is south.

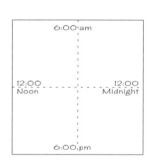

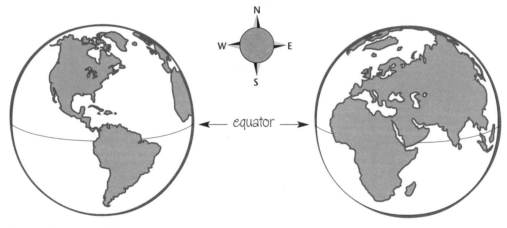

View of North and South America

equator

View of Eurasia and Africa

4. Straighten one of the loops of the paper clip. Tape the unbent half onto the center point of the folds of the paper.

5. Push the globe over the straight part of the paper clip, with the North Pole almost facing upward. Your model should look like the drawing to the right.

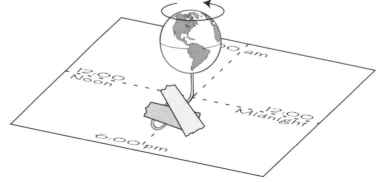

National Space Biomedical Research Institute
http://www.nsbri.org

From Outerspace to Innerspace / Sleep and Daily Rhythms
© 2000 Baylor College of Medicine

Activity 1

Day & Night

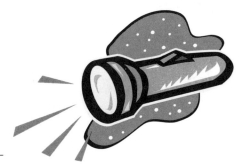

Name: _____

You will need:

Earth model that you constructed   Flashlight

You will use a flashlight to demonstrate how the sun shines toward Earth.

1. Hold the flashlight so that it points toward your Earth model along the marking for 12:00 noon.

2. Color a small dot on the Earth model that represents where you live. You will be observing what happens to this dot as the Earth model rotates.

3. Rotate the Earth model counterclockwise until the dot is at 6:00 a.m. This represents early morning in your locality. Notice where the sun (flashlight) is.

   Is the dot in the light or in the dark? _____

   Does the light shine directly toward the dot or to one side? _____

4. Rotate the Earth model 90 degrees (1/4 of a circle) in a counterclockwise direction. Notice where the sun (flashlight) is.

   Is the dot in the light or in the dark? _____

   Does the light shine directly toward the dot or to one side? _____

5. Rotate the Earth model another 90 degrees (1/4 of a circle). Notice where the sun (flashlight) is.

   Is the dot in the light or in the dark? _____

   Does the light shine directly toward the dot or to one side? _____

6. Rotate the Earth model another 90 degrees (1/4 of a circle). Notice where the sun (flashlight) is.

   Is the dot in the light or in the dark? _____

   Does the light shine directly toward the dot or to one side? _____

7. Based on your observations, write a short paragraph below describing why the sun appears overhead at noon, is visible in the western part of the sky in the evening and cannot be seen at midnight.

_____

_____

_____

CONCEPTS
- Many activities of living things occur in cycles of about 24 hours.
- Daily cycles are governed by internal "clocks."
- Internal clocks are cued by the environment, but run independently.

OVERVIEW
Students will observe that some behaviors and functions of living organisms vary predictably every 24 hours.

SCIENCE, HEALTH & MATH SKILLS
- Measuring
- Observing
- Drawing conclusions

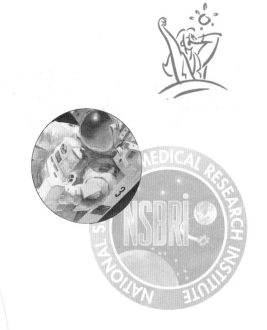

2. Living Clocks

Background

Most living things behave predictably in cycles of about 24 hours, similar to the period of the Earth's rotation. These cycles are referred to as *circadian*, from the Latin words for "about" (*circa*) and "day" (*dies*).

There are many easily recognized behavioral rhythms in nature. Well-known examples include the flowering of morning glories at dawn and the hunting routines of owls at night. These behaviors are governed by internal mechanisms, often referred to as "biological clocks," within the cells of the living organisms. When a biological clock runs on a 24-hour cycle, it also can be called a circadian clock.

Virtually all human body functions are governed by circadian clocks, such as waking and sleeping, body temperature (lower in the morning just after waking, higher in the afternoon), secretion of some hormones, and urine production. These changes occur regularly over intervals of 24 hours—without cues from the environment. Researchers once thought that, without cues from the environment, the human circadian clock eventually would drift into a slightly longer cycle of about 25 hours. More recent research has shown, however, that the free-running period of the human clock is just slightly over 24 hours in both young and older adults.

In this activity, students will explore daily cycles in themselves, animals and plants.

Time

Several 30-minute sessions, depending on the options selected

Materials

Materials will vary, depending on options selected.
- Source of natural sunlight
- Four bean plants per group (purchase or grow in small pots from seed)
- Fluorescent light (portable shop light or plant "grow light")
- One digital thermometer with several sterile covers per group
- Study animals (gerbil, bird, crickets, etc.)

Set-up and Management

Students should work in cooperative groups (2–4 students). Conduct discussions with the entire class.

Procedure

1. Have students work in collaborative groups to examine one or more of the following examples of daily cycles.

Body temperature. Have students measure the body temperature of each of the members of their group at three different times during the day over

In 1729, the French scientist Jean-Jacques de Mairan was the first to notice that the daily movements of the leaves of certain plants continued even when the plants were kept in constant dim light. Plants also have many other activities that vary according to the time of day. These activities include the opening of flowers, the release of fragrances, the opening and closing of pores in the leaves and the regulation of flowering at certain times of the year (determined by monitoring the length of darkness at night).

Activity 2
Body Temperature Data Sheet

several days. The times should be selected in advance and temperatures taken at the same time each day. For example, just after waking in the morning, eight hours later, and just before going to bed in the evening. Students can use a digital thermometer under the tongue (being sure to use a clean covering for each measurement) or a thermometer that they have at home. Measurements should be recorded as degrees F in a table like the one given on page 9. Have students calculate and graph the average temperature of the group

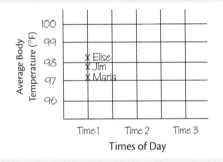

for each time of day. Ideally, students should make their first measurement just after waking and before eating or brushing their teeth. Similarly, for other measurements, students should wait at least 15 minutes after eating, drinking or brushing their teeth.

What students will observe: body temperature can be as much as 1–2 degrees lower in the very early morning than in the mid to late afternoon. This pattern is relatively consistent across individuals. Student results may not show this much change due to variations in body temperature caused by activity. Results also will be affected by the actual times at which temperature is measured.

Plant leaf movement. Grow young bean plants from seed or purchase them from a greenhouse. Plants grown from seed should have at

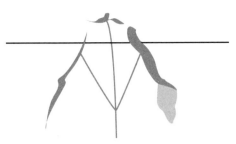

6:00 am
Bean leaves in the vertical position.

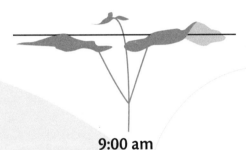

9:00 am
Bean leaves in the horizontal position.

least two leaves in addition to the cotyledons (fleshy seed leaves). Place the plants in a sunny window or in a growth chamber with a light timer, and have students note the orientation of the larger leaves as early as possible in the morning and again later in the afternoon. In particular, students should notice whether the leaves are extended outward or whether they are folded downward

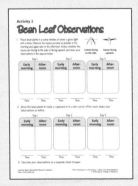

toward the stem. Have them repeat these observations over several days. Next, place the plants in a darkened corner of the room or cupboard, and have students observe and record the position of the leaves at the same times as before.

What students will observe: Leaves will be dropped toward the stem very early in the day and fully extended (horizontal) later in the day, regardless of whether the plants

Other plants show patterns of leaf movements similar to those that students observe in beans. The sensitive mimosa, kelanchoe, and wood sorrel are examples of plants that students can investigate.

The famous botanist, Carolus Linneaus, noticed that flowers of some plant species opened at predictable times of the day. Floral clocks, based on his idea, still are planted in parks and gardens. Traditionally, the "one o'clock" spot was planted with roses, "four o'clock" with hyacinths and "midnight," with pansies.

actually are exposed to the sun or artificial light.

Note. Students may observe that plants' stems curve toward the source of light. This movement is governed by chemicals inside the plant that cause cells on the side away from the light to lengthen more than cells on the side facing the light. This phenomenon is different from daily leaf movements, because it results in permanent changes in the shapes of the stems.

Animal behavior. If you have a hamster, or gerbil, with an exercise wheel in your classroom, have students observe and record the times of day when the rodent is active. Or have students observe and record the daily behaviors of other animals, such as fish, crickets (will chirp at approximately the same time each day) or birds, in the classroom. Students should record eating, resting and active times over several days to establish whether there is a predictable pattern to the animals' activities. Best results will be obtained if students make efforts to observe without disturbing their subjects and if light exposures are kept on a consistent schedule.

2. After students have concluded their investigations, have each group present its observations to the class. Students should be able to describe the behavior or body function that they observed, how they measured the behavior or function (by measuring temperature,

length of time spent on the exercise wheel, etc.) and the pattern or patterns that they discerned.

3. Discuss the results of the different investigations with the class. Ask questions to prompt students' thinking. *What did all of the cycles that you observed have in common? Did any of the patterns of behavior or function occur without the presence of normal sunlight? Do you think that something other than light is controlling the patterns that were observed?* Help students reach the conclusion that something inside each organism controls the observed patterns. Point out that most organisms have internal timers that regulate many aspects of their lives.

Variations

• The University of California-San Diego maintains a web site where students can monitor the daily behavior of a hamster,

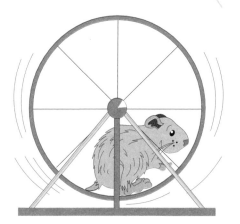

as well as check the hamster's behavior for the last few days. Have students log on at <http://varesearch.ucsd.edu/klem-fuss/sdhamstr.htm> and participate in the experiment.

Other cycles in living organisms are longer or shorter than 24 hours. Examples of longer cycles include fluctuation in levels of some human hormones (which vary predictably over several weeks), once-yearly flowering by many plants, and annual migration in a number of animal species. Shorter cycles include the cardiac cycle (heart beat) and the internal sleep cycle (stages of sleep).

_____

Because many body processes are rhythmic, the effectiveness of certain drugs or medicines will vary depending on the time of day.

Activity 2

Body Temperature Data Sheet

Record the body temperature (temp.) in °F of each member of your group three times each day. For best results, take the first reading just after waking in the morning and the third reading just before going to sleep at night. Wait at least 15 minutes after eating or drinking before you make a measurement.

Name

_____

Dates _____

_____

_____

_____

Morning—just after waking		Time during the day: _____		Evening—just before bed	
Time	Temp.	Time	Temp.	Time	Temp.

Name

_____

Dates _____

_____

_____

_____

Morning—just after waking		Time during the day: _____		Evening—just before bed	
Time	Temp.	Time	Temp.	Time	Temp.

Name

_____

Dates _____

_____

_____

_____

Morning—just after waking		Time during the day: _____		Evening—just before bed	
Time	Temp.	Time	Temp.	Time	Temp.

Name

_____

Dates _____

_____

_____

_____

Morning—just after waking		Time during the day: _____		Evening—just before bed	
Time	Temp.	Time	Temp.	Time	Temp.

On a separate sheet of paper, calculate the average temperature for each person at each time of day. Graph your results.

From Outerspace to Innerspace / Sleep and Daily Rhythms
© 2000 Baylor College of Medicine

National Space Biomedical Research Institute
http://www.nsbri.org

Activity 2

Bean Leaf Observations

1. Place bean plants in a sunny window, or under a grow light with a timer. Observe the leaves as early as possible in the morning and again later in the afternoon. Notice whether the leaves are facing to the side or facing upward, and draw your observations in the spaces below.

Leaves facing to the side.

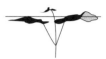

Leaves facing upward.

Day 1

Early morning	After-noon

_____ Time   _____ Time

Day 2

Early morning	After-noon

_____ Time   _____ Time

Day 3

Early morning	After-noon

_____ Time   _____ Time

2. Move the bean plants to inside a cupboard or to a dim corner of the room. Make your observations as before.

Day 1

Early morning	After-noon

_____ Time   _____ Time

Day 2

Early morning	After-noon

_____ Time   _____ Time

Day 3

Early morning	After-noon

_____ Time   _____ Time

3. Describe your observations on a separate sheet of paper.

National Space Biomedical Research Institute
http://www.nsbri.org

CONCEPTS
- All mammals, including humans, and many other kinds of animals need sleep.
- Most people have regular patterns of sleeping and waking.

OVERVIEW
Students will collect data about their own sleep patterns and, if desired, those of members of their families.

SCIENCE, HEALTH & MATH SKILLS
- Observation
- Data collection
- Graphing
- Drawing conclusions
- Learning to identify and practice healthy behaviors

3. Sleepy Time

Background

Sleep takes up about one-third of our lives. All mammals, including humans, and most vertebrates sleep. Many aspects of sleep still are not understood. Once viewed as passive shutting-down of most body systems, sleep now is known to consist of several stages, each with differing levels of brain and muscle activity.

Most of us sleep about the same number of hours and wake at about the same time each day, even without an alarm. Many, however, vary their sleep patterns using external alarm clocks to meet school or work schedules. Daily wake-up times in humans are governed by an internal clock, consisting of about 10,000 nerve cells located deep inside the brain. Even without any light or sound cues, most people sleep and wake in cycles of close to 24 hours.

Patterns of sleeping and waking vary by age. For instance, newborns sleep 16–18 hours each day, including several naps. By age one, children sleep 12–14 hours, including about two naps. Nine or ten hours of sleep, without naps, is normal for children by age 12. Adults sleep about eight hours per day. The urge to nap in the afternoon is normal for teenagers and adults, and most override this urge to sleep by remaining active. For some who may be in a sleep-promoting setting, a nap may occur with possible hazardous consequences.

Time

30 minutes to conduct initial class discussion; 3–7 days for students to collect data on sleep times; 30 minutes for discussion of results

Materials

Each student will need:
- Log or journal
- Copies of *Sleeping Patterns Graph* on page 13

Set-up and Management

Begin the activity with a discussion involving the entire class. Working individually, students will collect data on themselves and family members. They will share their results with other members of their groups.

Procedure

1. Challenge students to think about all the different things that they do every day. Let each student suggest one or more activities and create a list on the board.

2. Now ask, *What activities could you leave out of this list without affecting your health or how you feel? What activities must stay on the list? Why do you think so?*

3. Explain to students that they will be examining one of the essential activities on the list—sleep. Encourage students to share what they know

All animals rest between periods of activity. Sleep patterns vary among different animals. Rabbits, for example, sleep for only a few minutes at a time. Dolphins have a unique form of sleeping: one half of the dolphin brain sleeps, while the other half continues to be alert and wide awake.

about sleep. For instance, *when do they usually sleep, how long do they sleep, what makes them wake?*

4. Have each student create a journal, or "Sleep Log," to record the times he or she goes to sleep and wakes daily. The journal should include: waking time; how student felt at waking; how student felt during the day (tired, well rested, etc.); bed time; and how student felt at bedtime. If possible, time the activity so that students are able to compare weeknight and weekend sleep patterns. Students may want to ask other members of their families to participate and record their family members' data as well.

5. After 3–5 days, have students graph their data on the *Sleeping Patterns Graph.* Also have students calculate the average number of hours of sleep received by each person included in the study.

Activity 3
Sleeping Patterns Graph

6. Have students share and compare their graphs and journals with other members of their groups. Help them look for similarities and differences.

Also help the students identify patterns in their graphs. Ask questions such as, *Do most people go to bed and wake up at about the same time each day? Did you feel particularly sleepy on any day during this activity? Why or why not? Can you notice anything different about the part of the graph corresponding to that day? Who sleeps more—children or grown-ups? What about very young children—do they have the same sleep patterns as older children or adults?*

Variations

*   In addition to recording sleeping and waking times, also have students record other essential activities, such as eating or exercising, in their journals.

*   Have students investigate the sleeping habits of different kinds of animals (*Where do they sleep and for how long?*, etc.).

*   Have students create a sheet of paper with 24 squares by folding it in half three times, followed by folding it into thirds. Have them number the squares with the hours of the day. Next, ask students to draw the activity that they did most during each hour of the day in the corresponding square. Have them count the number of squares dedicated to sleeping, eating, playing, studying, etc.

Scientists only are beginning to understand why we sleep and what happens when we sleep. Sleep consists of two different phases. One phase, called non-REM sleep, is characterized by slow brain activity, no eye movement and lack of muscle tone. Another phase, Rapid Eye-Movement (REM) sleep, is characterized by an active brain, bursts of eye movements, and paralyzed muscles (which makes it safe to dream!).

Dreams are prevalent during REM sleep. Scientists have different ideas about why we dream. Some believe that the brain consolidates needed and erases unneeded information during dreaming.

Activity 3

Sleeping Patterns Graph

Color in the square representing your bed time and the square corresponding to your wake time for each day recorded in your journal. Use a different color to fill in the squares between the bed and wake times. Record days of the week and hours slept.

Day of the Week	Hours Slept
_____	_____
_____	_____
_____	_____
_____	_____
_____	_____
_____	_____

Noon
11 am
10 am
9 am
8 am
7 am
6 am
5 am
4 am
3 am
2 am
1 am
Midnight
11 pm
10 pm
9 pm
8 pm
7 pm
6 pm

| Day | Day | Day | Day | Day | Day | Day |

From Outerspace to Innerspace / Sleep and Daily Rhythms
© 2000 Baylor College of Medicine

National Space Biomedical Research Institute
http://www.nsbri.org

- Sleeping and waking are governed by an internal clock.
- The internal "sleep" clock is influenced by external cues.
- Changes in schedules can conflict with the body's internal clock.

OVERVIEW
Students will investigate the effects of changing their bedtimes on their sleep patterns.

SCIENCE, HEALTH & MATH SKILLS
- Predicting
- Observing
- Drawing conclusions

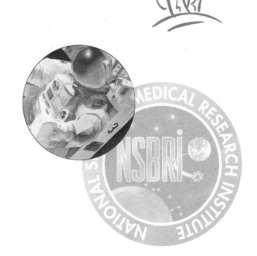

4. I've Got Rhythm

Background

As students discovered previously, most people go to sleep and wake up at about the same times each day. This sleep cycle is regulated inside the brain by a group of nerve cells that govern sleeping and waking. These cells, which act as a timer, or "biological clock," stay atuned to the outside environment by receiving time cues. Sunlight, a strong time cue, is detected by the retina (the part of the eye that has receptors for light), which sends messages to the brain. Daily exposure to light keeps the body's sleep cycle synchronized to conditions outside.

Abrupt changes in sleeping times, such as that due to air travel or a change in work schedule, can cause difficulty with falling asleep or staying awake, because external cues conflict with messages being sent by the body's internal clock. The brain may be signaling *sleep,* while outside conditions may be saying *be active, it's morning!* It can take several days to adjust to a new time zone. Other factors also can affect the sleep cycle. For example, physical exercise, medicines, meal times and stimulants, (such as caffeine in coffee, tea and soft drinks).

This activity allows students to investigate their own internal clocks. Students will try going to bed one hour earlier than usual and observe the effects that it has on their abilities to fall asleep immediately and on their waking times the next morning.

Time

30–60 minutes to conduct initial class discussion; 30–60 minutes to summarize findings on the following day

Materials

Each student will need:
- copy of *Sleep Observations* page

Set-up and Management

Conduct discussions of the activity with the entire class. Students will carry out their own investigations at home and report back the following day.

Procedure

Day One

1. Remind students of the results of the previous activities. *Did the leaves of the bean plants move in the same way each day? How about the animals that were observed? Did their behavior show a daily pattern? Do you also do things at about the same time each day?* Have students refer to the sleep journals they created. *Do you think some of the things you do are controlled by an internal clock?*

2. Explain to students that they will be investigating their own biological clocks for sleeping and waking. For one night, they will change their bedtime to one hour earlier than usual, and observe what happens.

3. Mention the types of observations

A group of nerve cells that act as a biological clock was first located in the brains of house sparrows. Biological clocks now have been identified in vertebrates, such as mammals, reptiles and some amphibians—and even invertebrates, such as fruit flies, cockroaches, crickets and mollusks. "Clocks" also have been found in single-celled organisms, like mold and bacteria.

Teenagers often have a sleep cycle that is shifted so that their internally programmed sleeping time ends up beginning around midnight. This may make it difficult for them to get enough sleep if they do not regulate light exposure carefully.

that students will make. For example, they should note whether it was easy or hard to fall asleep at the earlier time and whether they woke at their usual times the next morning. Students also should notice how they felt the next day—more sleepy, less sleepy, etc.

4. Distribute copies of the student sheets on which students should record their observations. Explain to students that individual results will vary from person to person. If possible, have each student enlist the help of a parent or older brother or sister to record the actual time that the student falls asleep.

Day Two

1. Have students summarize their observations by writing a short paragraph about how they felt as they tried to go to sleep at an earlier time. Stimulate their thinking by asking questions, such as, *Was it easier or more difficult than usual to go to sleep at a new time? Did you notice noises and other people more or less? How did you feel the next morning? Did you wake at your usual time?*

2. Have students share their paragraphs with the rest of the class by reading them aloud or by posting them somewhere in the classroom. Initiate a class discussion of the results. Point out that some students may have had difficulty falling asleep early because their bodies were used to sleeping at a later time. Likewise, students may have woken at their usual times in the morning, even after receiving an extra hour of sleep, because of the programming of their internal clocks.

3. You may find that some students feel better after receiving the extra sleep. Initiate a discussion of how much sleep is typically obtained by children (see page 11) and how lack of sleep can impair performance on both mental and physical tasks. For example, lack of sleep, like alcohol intoxication, can make physical reactions slower.

Variations

- Have students continue with the earlier bedtimes for several days. *Do they eventually become used to the earlier times?*

- Invite another teacher or a parent who has traveled across several time zones (across the continental US or to Europe, for example) to talk to the class about how he or she felt physically for the first one or two days in the new location. *Was it easy to sleep? Did he or she have to make adjustments again after returning home?*

- Invite a policeman, fireman or someone else who routinely works a night shift to talk to the class about how he or she has adapted to the stresses of a nocturnal work schedule.

- Some animals are more active at night than during the day. Have students investigate examples of nocturnal animals (bats, owls, luna moths, etc.) and report back to the class. *What advantages might a nocturnal lifestyle have for different kinds of animals?*

Sleep disorders affect up to 70 million people in the US. Insomnia is a sleep disorder which causes people to have difficulty staying asleep. Apnea is a disorder in which people have difficulty breathing while asleep.

Astronauts frequently have difficulty sleeping. This may be because their internal clocks are not synchronized to the light conditions they experience. In addition, the stresses of space flight and hectic work schedules can affect the quality of astronauts' sleep. Researchers are looking for ways to address these problems in space. Their results will help many people on Earth with sleep disorders.

In many places in the US, everyone sets their clocks ahead one hour in the Spring and leaves them that way until the Fall. Switching to Daylight Savings Time can cause temporary adjustment problems for some people because their sleeping times are changed by one hour.

Activity 4

Sleep Observations

You will need to ask a family member or friend to help with this experiment.

You will be going to bed one hour earlier than usual. Write your observations in the spaces below.

1. What time did you go to bed? _____

2. What time did you fall asleep? (Have someone write this down for you.) _____

3. How did you feel when you went to bed early? _____

4. What time did you wake the next morning? _____

5. How did you feel the next morning? _____

6. In class, write a paragraph about your experiment in the space below.

_____

_____

_____

_____

_____

_____

_____

_____

_____

_____

Name _____

CONCEPTS
• Time can be measured using the relative positions of the Earth and sun.

OVERVIEW
Students will make a sundial (shadow clock) and use it to tell time.

SCIENCE, HEALTH & MATH SKILLS
• Measuring
• Locating cardinal directions
• Making a model
• Observing
• Drawing conclusions

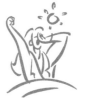

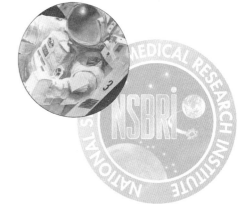

5. Shifting Shadows

Background

For a very long time, people relied on the position of the sun in the sky to estimate the time of day. Noon or midday was designated as the time when the sun was at its highest point. We now know, of course, that the sun does not move across the sky as it appears. Rather, the Earth rotates as it revolves around the sun.

One of the earliest ways of measuring time used the predictable changes in shadows that occurred as the sun moved across the sky. Since shadows change predictably over the course of each day, they can be used to estimate time. A stick placed vertically in the ground probably was the first sundial. Simple sundials were used to tell time in Egypt more than 3,000 years ago.

In early times, an hour was calculated as 1/12 of the period of daylight. Thus, depending on the time of year, the length of the hours in the day varied. Now, we divide each day into 24 equal hours, which remain unchanged regardless of the time of year. Today, time also is standardized from place to place. Before 1884, every locality set its clocks to the highest position of the sun (=noon). This led to considerable confusion, because every town ran on a different time. Now, the world is sectioned into 24 standard time zones that are uniform. Each time zone accounts for 15 degrees longitude and 60 minutes of Universal Time.

Time

10 minutes for set-up; two 30–45 minute periods to conduct activity

Materials

Each group will need:
• flashlight
• paper plate
• coffee stirrer
• permanent marker
• compass

Set-up and Management

Place the materials in a central area for Materials Managers to collect for their groups. Have students work in groups of four to conduct the activity.

Procedure

Day One

1. Ask students to observe while you use a flashlight and your hand to make a shadow. Turn the light source off, then ask *Where is the shadow?* Students should understand that when an object is in front of a light source, it blocks the light, causing an area of darkness—a shadow. Encourage students to "play" with light and shadows using the flashlights.

2. Challenge students to think about what happens to shadows outdoors as the position of the sun changes relative to the Earth's surface. Ask questions such as, *Are shadows always the same size? Why or why not? When are shadows outside smallest? When are*

Over the course of history, different civilizations explained the cycle of night and day in different ways. For example, some ancient priests of India believed the Earth to be supported on 12 huge pillars. At night time, the sun was believed to pass underneath.

Aristotle, a Greek philosopher, was certain that the entire sky revolved around the Earth. This Earth-centered view of the universe was prevalent in Europe until the 16th century.

Copernicus, a Polish clergyman and scientist, is credited with providing the world with a new theory of the solar system, in which planets (including Earth) revolve around the sun.

they largest? Can we always see shadows outside? Have students think about whether there is a pattern to the sizes of shadows made by the sun (shadows are longest in the morning and evening, and shortest at mid-day). Using flashlights and pencils, have students make shadows of different lengths. Ask them to identify variables that affect the length of the shadows.

3. Challenge students to consider whether there is a pattern to the way the positions of shadows change over the course of a day. *Do shadows stay in the same place all day?* Explain to students that they will be investigating patterns in shadow movement. They will be using the patterns they discover to solve a practical problem: telling time.

4. Distribute copies of the Shadow Clock sheet on page 19 to students. Following the instructions given on the sheet for Day One, they will work in groups to create Shadow Clocks (sundials).

5. Note that if the observations are made during normal school hours, the clocks will be calibrated only for a portion of the total day. As an alternative, consider having students also calibrate their Shadow Clocks at home, so that the clocks will be useful for the full range of daylight.

Day Two

1. Students will use their Shadow Clocks in a new location and compare times of day, as measured by their Shadow Clocks, to times shown by a watch or clock. Each group must use a compass to orient their Shadow Clocks in the same direction as on Day One.

2. After students have completed both days' activities, conduct a discussion

about the accuracy of the Shadow Clocks. Ask, *How well did your Shadow Clocks measure time, as compared to a watch or clock? Why do you think the Shadow Clocks did (or did not) measure time as accurately as the other clocks?* Also, ask students to consider when the Shadow Clocks might not be useful. Examples: night-time (too dark), when skies are cloudy (no shadows), at different times of the year (shadow pattern will be different, so clocks might not predict time correctly), in different locations (pattern will change if other location is at a different latitude).

3. Brainstorm with students on ways to improve the Shadow Clocks. Have them look on the Internet or in the library to find other sundials.

Variations

• Have students try using shadow length to predict the time.

• Have students think about why time zones that account for a one-hour time difference are separated by 15° of longitude.

• Using a globe or an atlas, have students figure out what time it would be in London, Los Angeles, Honolulu and Moscow, if it were 8:00 a.m. in St. Louis, Missouri.

• To learn more about sundials, have students check the NASA Web site at <http://liftoff.msfc.nasa.gov/acad-emy/earth/sundial/sundial-how.html>.

STANDARD TIME

Coordinated Universal Time (UTC) formerly Greenwich Mean Time (GMT)

W to E subtract 24 hours

E to W add 24 hours

International Date Line (approximately)

In 1972, Universal Time replaced Greenwich Mean Time as the standard reference for telling time. Universal Time, also referred to as International Atomic Time, is measured by an atomic clock. The atomic clock uses the extremely regular vibrations that occur within atoms to measure time.

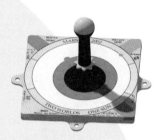

A sundial based on drawings from children across the US will travel to Mars aboard NASA's Mars Surveyor 2001 lander. Inscribed with the words "Two Worlds, One Sun," the sundial will be 3 inches (about 8 cm) square, and weigh just over 2 ounces (60 grams).
Image courtesy of NASA.

The position that the sun appears to have in the sky depends on where you are on the Earth's surface.

Activity 5

Shadow Clock

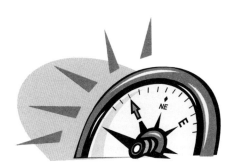

Your group will need:

Disposable paper plate

Coffee stirrer

Compass

Permanent marker

DAY ONE

1. Turn the plate upside down and write the letter "N" on one edge of the plate to mark the side that should face North.

2. With the plate still turned upside-down, make a very small hole in the center using the tip of a pencil. Push the coffee stirrer through the plate about one-half to one inch. Put the plate back on the table. The stirrer should "stand" straight up.

3. Take the plate outside and place it in a sunny place.

4. Using the compass, position the plate so that the "N" is facing North. (If it is windy outside, you may need to tape the plate down).

5. Using the marker, carefully trace the line created by the shadow of the coffee stirrer on the plate and label the time as shown above.

6. At one-hour intervals, repeat steps 4–5.

7. After you have made as many one-hour readings as possible, bring your Shadow Clock back inside.

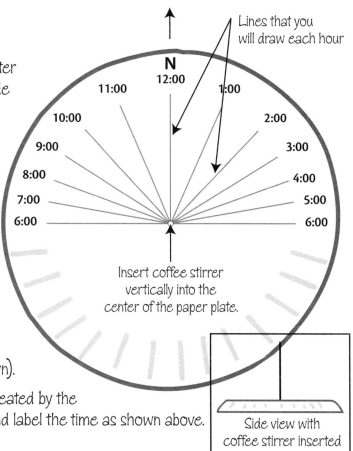

Lines that you will draw each hour

Insert coffee stirrer vertically into the center of the paper plate.

Side view with coffee stirrer inserted

DAY TWO

1. Now you will test the accuracy of your Shadow Clock. Take the clock outside to a new location.

2. Use a compass to position the plate so that the "N" is facing North.

3. Observe where the shadow line falls on the plate. Based on the markings you already have made, estimate the current time as accurately as possible.

4. Compare your estimate to the time as measured by a watch or clock. How close were you?

5. On a separate sheet, describe why the Shadow Clock worked or didn't work. Does the Shadow Clock have any advantages over a mechanical clock? Does it have any disadvantages?

CONCEPTS
- Many different factors affect the quality of sleep.
- Astronauts traveling in space experience many disruptions of normal sleep patterns.

OVERVIEW
Language arts activity in which students brainstorm about when they have had difficulty sleeping, read about how astronauts sleep in space, and write about unusual places in which they have slept.

SCIENCE, HEALTH & MATH SKILLS
- Identifying common elements
- Making extensions to new situations

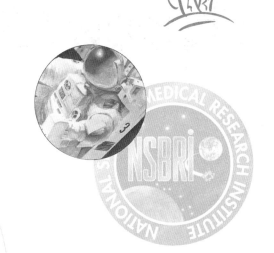

6. Sleeping in Space

Background

Many different factors can affect the quality of sleep. All of us have had difficulty sleeping at one time or another. Excitement, anxiety or stress, consumption of stimulants, unusual surroundings, noises, travel across time zones, or changes in daily schedules can make sleeping difficult. Insomnia is the word used to describe an ongoing inability to get enough sleep to feel rested during the day. More than 50% of Americans suffer from occasional bouts of insomnia or other sleep disorders.

Astronauts probably experience more disruptions of normal sleep patterns than anyone else. The intense work schedule, unusual surroundings, cramped work quarters, stress and excitement of being in space all can make sleeping difficult. Space motion sickness also can contribute to sleeping problems. In addition, the normal 24-hour pattern of light and darkness that provides a time cue to the body's internal sleeping and waking cycle is absent.

Since lack of sleep can seriously affect performance on physical and mental tasks, helping astronauts overcome sleeping problems is a priority. Several days before launching into space, crew members are exposed to bright lights at specific times, a controlled environment and programmed meal periods to help reset their bodies' internal clocks to match the schedules that will be followed in space. Research to help astronauts sleep better also helps people on Earth with similar problems.

Time

10 minutes for set-up; 30–60 minutes to conduct activity

Materials

Each student or group of students will need:
- Copies of student pages *Catching Zzzzz's* and *Are You Sleeping?*

Set-up and Management

Conduct this activity with the entire class. Students may read the story, *Catching Zzzzz's*, individually, or they make work in teams.

Procedure

1. Ask students to remember an occasion when they had difficulty sleeping. Have them share their experiences with the rest of the class, and list the experiences on the board or on an overhead. Scenarios suggested by students might include: the night before an exciting event, such as a birthday party; trying to sleep in the car during a long trip; or being wakened by strange or frightening noises at night.

2. Encourage students to think carefully about the list and to identify common elements among the events. Such elements could include: sleeping in places other than home; sleeping before or after unusual events; sleeping when one's physical state is not normal

Students can do several things to make sure they will be rested and ready to perform well in school.

- Avoid soft drinks or foods with caffeine (for example, chocolate, some soft drinks, coffee, tea).

- Stick to a regular schedule for going to bed and waking up, and get some bright light in the morning.

- Get some light exercise in the late afternoon (but not in the evening before going to bed).

- Recognize that, on average, most students need at least nine to ten hours of sleep per night, and plan schedules accordingly.

(sick with an itchy rash, etc.).

3. Mention to students that they will be reading about how astronauts sleep in space. Ask, *Do you think astronauts can sleep as well in space as they can at home? What might be different about sleeping in space?* After students have offered their comments, distribute copies of the *Catching Zzzzz's* and *Are You Sleeping?* pages.

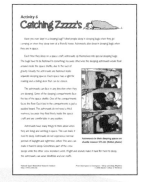

4. Students may read the essay and complete the reading and writing extensions on their own or by working together in small groups.

5. Provide an opportunity for students to share their work by having them read the paragraphs that they created as part of the writing activity on page 23, or by displaying the paragraphs somewhere in class.

Variations

• Have students create drawings to accompany their paragraphs on sleeping.

• Encourage students to access NASA-associated sites on the World Wide Web. NASA's homepage is a good place to start <www.nasa.gov>.

• Encourage students to find out about other occupations in which the sleeping circumstances might be unusual.

Why do we sleep? Scientists still are investigating this question. Some people believe that sleep helps the body recover from activities during waking hours and also helps in the formation of memories. Some animals also might sleep to save energy during hours when it is too dark or too dangerous to hunt for food.

Sleeplessness diminishes mental and physical performance. In addition, a sleepy body is more susceptible to the effects of drugs and alcohol. Sleepiness can build up day, after day, after day, creating a sleep "debt" that may be hard to "pay back."

Activity 6
Catching Zzzzz's

Have you ever slept in a sleeping bag? Most people sleep in sleeping bags when they go camping or when they sleep over at a friend's house. Astronauts also sleep in sleeping bags when they are in space.

Each time they sleep on a space craft, astronauts zip themselves into special sleeping bags. The bags have to be fastened to something, because otherwise the sleeping astronauts would float around inside the space shuttle, due to the lack of gravity. Usually, the astronauts are fastened inside separate sleeping spaces. Each space has a light for reading and a sliding door that can be closed.

The astronauts can face in any direction when they are sleeping. Some of the sleeping compartments face the top of the space shuttle. One of the compartments faces the floor. Each bed in the compartments is just a padded board. The astronauts do not need a thick mattress, because they float freely inside the space craft and are comfortable in any position.

Astronauts have many things to think about when they are living and working in space. This can make it hard to sleep. Astronauts do not experience normal periods of daylight and night time, either. This also can make it hard to sleep. Sometimes, part of the crew sleeps while the other crew members work. If light and sounds make it hard for them to sleep, the astronauts can wear blindfolds and ear muffs.

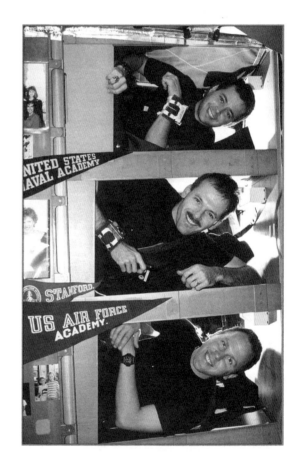

Astronauts in their sleeping spaces on shuttle mission STS-68. (NASA photo)

Activity 6

Are You Sleeping?

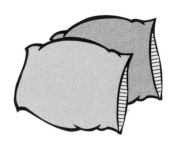

1. Make a list of the ways in which sleeping in space is just like sleeping on Earth.

_____

_____

_____

_____

_____

_____

_____

2. Make a list of the ways in which sleeping in space is different from sleeping on Earth.

_____

_____

_____

_____

_____

_____

_____

3. In the space below or on a separate sheet, write a paragraph about the most unusual place in which you ever slept. Include answers to the following questions: Where did you sleep? How well did you sleep? Would you like to sleep there every day?

_____

_____

_____

_____

_____

_____

_____

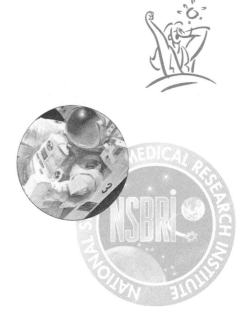

CONCEPTS
- Many organisms show daily cycles of activities or functions.
- Daily cycles (also called circadian rhythms) are about 24 hours long—the same as one rotation of the Earth.
- Circadian rhythms in living things are controlled by internal biological clocks that are set to local environmental conditions.
- The timing of when humans sleep and wake is governed by an internal clock.
- People can have difficulty sleeping if external conditions change suddenly and no longer agree with the settings of their internal clocks.

OVERVIEW
Summative/assessment activity: students will review concepts about sleep and daily cycles using a fun poem, and will create their own illustrated rhymes.

SCIENCE, HEALTH & MATH SKILLS
- Integrating information
- Drawing conclusions

7. Twenty-Four Hours a Day

Background
Cycles and rhythms can be found in all organisms on Earth. Many of these cycles are synchronized to the 24-hour cycle of the Earth's rotation about its axis.

The timing of when people are asleep and awake is determined to a large extent by an internal clock. Environmental cues, particularly light, keep the clock synchronized to external conditions. The clock itself, however, will continue to run on approximate 24-hour cycles, even without changes in the environment.

The human cycle of sleeping and waking can become disrupted if external conditions, particularly light, change. This happens when travelers move across time zones or when astronauts travel in space.

Space life scientists are looking for ways to help astronauts achieve the sleep they need to function well under the stresses of long-term space flight. Their research also will help solve sleep-related problems for people on Earth.

Time
10 minutes for set-up; 45 minutes to conduct activity

Materials
Each student or group will need:
- copy of *Tick-Tock, Tick-Tock*, page 26
- paper to create a poem
- markers, crayons, etc., to illustrate new poem

Set-up and Management
Conduct a summary discussion of the major concepts in the unit by reciting the poem on page 26 with the class. Students should work independently or in small groups for the remainder of the activity.

Procedure
1. Review the major concepts to which students were exposed in this unit, as outlined in the Background section of this activity.

2. Read or have students read the poem, *Tick-Tock, Tick-Tock*. Talk about the concepts in the poem.

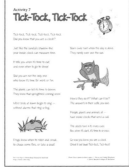

3. Have students create their own

illustrated poems. Several options are possible.

- Distribute the poem to students.
- After reading the poem, let students write their own poems on sleep and biological clocks; or
- Read a few of the verses to get students started, and then suggest that they write verses of their own to complete the poem; or
- Share the first few lines of each verse and have the students complete the verses with their own inspirations; or
- Devise your own way to inspire students to express their knowledge about biological rhythms and clocks in verse.

Activity 7
Tick-Tock, Tick-Tock

Tick-tock, Tick-tock, Tick-tock, Tick-tock.
Did you know that you are a clock?

Just like the sundial's shadow-line
your inside clock can measure time.

It tells you when it's time to eat,
and even when to go to sleep!

But you are not the only one
who know it's time for work or fun.

The plants can tell it's time to bloom.
They know that springtime's coming soon!

Most birds at dawn begin to sing —
without alarms that ring-a-ling.

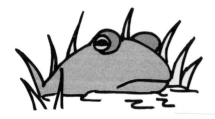

Frogs know when to ribbit and croak,
to chase some flies, or take a soak!

Barn owls hunt when the day is done.
They rarely ever see the sun.

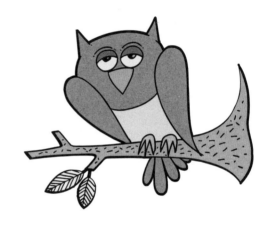

How'd they do it? What can it be?
The answer's in their cells, you see.

People, plants and animals all —
have inside clocks that send a call.

The clocks tune in to many cues
like, when it's dark, it's time to snooze.

So now you know you are a clock,
Shout it out loud: Tick-tock, Tick-tock!

National Space Biomedical Research Institute
http://www.nsbri.org